Your Body Retain the Score

The body and soul of Relieving Trauma

By

Gold M. Crown

Table of contents

Introduction

The Discovery of Trauma

What is Trauma?

The phrase **"trauma"** is used to describe experiences or conditions which are emotionally painful and distressing, and that crush people's ability to manage, leaving them powerless. Trauma has every so often been defined in connection with circumstances that might be outdoor the world of normal humans revel. Unfortunately, this definition doesn't always maintain genuinely. For some organizations of humans, trauma can occur regularly and emerge as a part of the commonplace human experience. Trauma also method different things relying on wherein it's miles used. It can discuss a mind injury in medical settings, an existence-threatening occasion in intellectual fitness settings, or a scary/distressing experience in social settings.

Traumatic occasions that take place as both kids and adults can cause permanent changes in our psychological and physical responses to stress. The period 'trauma' describes any unexpected circumstance in which someone's emotional or physical well-being is disturbed by using the strain of the scenario. Any scenario can bring about trauma, even though not unusual examples consist of:

- Witnessing demise
- Emotional forgetting or abuse
- Physical injury
- Natural screw ups

Once an annoying occasion has befallen, it's miles regular and wholesome for someone to enjoy grief or unhappiness for a positive period. However, some humans increase distressing signs and symptoms that persist for longer than they need to. These signs become overwhelming to someone's ability to stay an everyday and healthy existence. Additionally, the signs do not appear to ease or wane as time goes on.

What are unique styles of trauma?

Trauma could have a huge effect on your life. Everyone experiences something radical every so often, but if you have not been capable of giving it a place yet, we're talking about trauma. Trauma treatment is superb help that can make recuperation less difficult and quicker.

Types of trauma:

Dungeon trauma

In loss trauma, the individual loses something or someone irreplaceable and extraordinarily precious or cherished.

Loss of a cherished one by using the loss of life, for instance, if dad and mom, brother or sister die.

Loss of a cherished one as a result of divorce, for instance for kids while their dad and mom divorce, once they must be admitted to a medical institution or social services as kids, or while their own family individuals separate due to a struggling state of affairs.

Loss of elements or functions of one's own body due to an accident or infection.

Loss of fabric assets, inclusive of loss of a residence due to natural disaster or fire, loss of home and home due to struggle or expulsion from the homeland.

Empathic trauma

Personal harm, on the whole, involves an unmarried person, including a motorcyclist who has an extreme twist of fate or someone who almost drowns whilst swimming.

Spectators of a trauma scenario also can end up traumatized, that is, critically stunned, panicked, and emotionally stressed for the long term any more.

Group trauma

In many cases, several humans or groups of humans had been involved in a disturbing state of affairs, together with an automobile coincidence or a bank theft. Due to the not unusual trauma, the survivors turn out to be a group of struggling colleagues.

Such businesses, therefore, develop a commonplace identification as victims and survivors, although they did not realize each other earlier. Examples are conflict veterans or plane crash survivors.

Family trauma

This is a trauma that happens in a collection of individuals who belong together through blood dating or marriage.

A worrying occasion in an own family circle is, for example, the surprising death of a figure or child, the abduction of a baby, the surprising unemployment of their own family supporter, the unexpected termination of the hire of a residence, the separation from their own family due to battle.

Family trauma may have a long-lasting effect on family contributors.

Ethnic trauma

We speak about ethnic trauma when greater humans are affected who merge as a set into a bigger network and express this in a not unusual language, in customs and rituals, in faith and livelihood.

National Trauma

In the case of national trauma, fate strikes a country or a whole people. There are five groups of causes:

Natural disasters include earthquakes, floods, drought, and bloodlessness.

Technical disasters, such as a catastrophe at a nuclear energy plant.

Economic screw-ups, including foreign money depreciation.

Terror: prepared violence to gain a specific aim, usually political

War.

Emotional and psychological trauma: is the result of relatively demanding activities that shatter your feeling of protection, making you experience helplessness and inclined in a risky global environment.

These many uses make trauma a tough phrase to define.

Let's discuss trauma as it pertains to mental fitness.

Below, are provided numerous more unique terms that get at various aspects of psychological trauma.

Traumatic occasion:

An event that threatens our sense of bodily or mental protection. It is often perceived as life-threatening. Examples of trauma include physical/emotional abuse, sexual attack/rape, combat/battle, motor automobile injuries, or natural disasters.

Traumatic Stress:

Our frame's response to an annoying occasion. Experiencing an annoying event triggers a pressure response in our mind's alarm device, releasing cortisol and other stress hormones
The strain reaction is often referred to as the "combat, flight, or freeze reaction."
It keeps us alive and signals us of risk.
When we revel in an occasion that our brain perceives as existence threatening, other components of our brain shut down. This permits us to react fast and mechanically, which

includes getting out of the way of an oncoming automobile.

This is an everyday, adaptive response to trauma. Mostly, our brains work properly. However, in a few events, or with repeated publicity to trauma, our brains can **"rewire,"** leading to extra continual demanding strain symptoms, such as PTSD

In PTSD, the alarm structures of our brain become overactive, tricking us into believing that we're in danger even if no danger exists.

Posttraumatic Stress Disorder (PTSD:

A scientific analysis for humans experiencing the following forms of trauma signs: feeling constantly on the aspect, averting matters that remind us of the occasion, having unwanted mind or memories associated with the event (e.G., flashbacks), problems controlling our mood, or having nightmares of the occasion.

A PTSD analysis will now not be made until signs and symptoms have persisted for at least one month after the traumatic occasion.

About thirteen% of those who experience a demanding occasion go directly to increase PTSD, however, the chance of developing PTSD increases with higher ranges of trauma publicity. With sufficient trauma publicity, we would all in all likelihood expand PTSD.

Evidence shows that PTSD signs and symptoms will now not go away on their personal.

Fortunately, numerous treatment options exist and have been proven to be powerful in reducing PTSD signs and symptoms, along with extended exposure (PE), eye motion desensitization and reprocessing remedy (EMDR), trauma targeted CBT, and narrative publicity therapy.

If you've experienced a worrying event and suspect you have got PTSD, discover a certified mental fitness expert with information on treating trauma/PTSD.

What's thrilling is that the same occasion might be awful but no longer soul-wounding the first time, but soul-wounding on a subsequent prevalence. Torment can be like that for a while, it's simply fooling around, then oneday antagonistically hollows into you with real enmity, no person allows you, and your soul receives snick.

A lot of traumatized human beings are very careworn. They sense despair and tension and experience that something from their beyond is inflicting it, but due to the fact they can discover a major annoying episode (like being mugged and crushed up), they think not anything awful occurred to them.

What passed off to them turned into continual, now not acute, trauma. Torment, Separation, war in the family, child abuse and negletion, and displeasing family dynamics. Because it became their ordinary development, they don't perceive it as abnormal. Eventually, tension and/or despair develop, and they don't recognize why. Our minds try to protect us and maintain us from confronting emotional ache that is backlogged in our brains. The individuals who deny they have got it the most vigorously are often those who have it the most deeply.

Chapter 1

Understanding the thoughts and the mind

Neuroscience does not restrict the mind to the mind but understands it as a whole body experience. For example, our peripheral nervous system largely creates our feel of self and presence via visceral feedback from muscle tissue and proprioception that defines the bounds, shape, and movement capacity of the body. The mind has no lifestyles impartial of the frame aside from in dreaming, and goals are a pale replacement for the arena, for they handiest toss round pictures gleaned from the sector in waking. Every machine is encouraged via the brain feeds that impact the lower back upon the mind. It is a two-man road. Even the thoughts jogging through our heads turn out to be ideomotor twitches of the larynx in preparation for speech. The brain may organize the speech behavior and repress its full expression, but the experience of thinking, what you'll name the intellectual qualia of idea-speech, is inseparable from the vocal apparatus and the breath. Like this, a maximum of the mind's methods appear at an unconscious level. We turn out to be aware of them; they enter our minds best as they advantage a few shapes of physical expression.

This perspective, that the body creates the mind as an epiphenomenon, is Materialism, frequently referred to as Realism. The opponent's philosophy is that of Idealism. Here, the valuable idea is that we can not prove that the frame creates the mind due to the fact ideas themselves are born of thoughts. In different words, the thoughts are primary. It takes a mind to understand and understand that there is also a frame. Visionaries move one step farther and say there may be no evidence that the complete world, body and all, isn't contained inside the mind, and that truth isn't an illusion like a dream. The Naturalist argues that the body should be number one due to the fact that whilst the body dies, so do the thoughts. The visionary wonders how the naturalist knows this as fact without being departed.

Visionaries and Naturalists each have their absurd extremes. Solipsists declare that the complete world is an illusion and the person's thoughts are the best real aspect that exists. Whereas s declare the exceptional global is just a painting of the hidden international, solipsists deny even the hidden international. On the other extreme are the 'naive' naturalists, who are so materialistic they deny that the mind exists altogether, and could even deny that existence is occurring properly now inside the moment. For them, theoretical bodies strolling the crust of a theoretical spinning rock is the final truth, and the actuality of it in enjoyment is just a confounding variable to be ignored. Both extremes border on ridiculousness, as they each in their very own manner deny life. We nonetheless have no longer observed a way around Descartes' fundamental observation that the very fact we're capable of contemplating the question approach that there exists a mind to do the brooding about.

So from the philosophical fork in the street, we appear down both paths that seem on the outset to guide in contrary instructions and see that they each cause the identical useless cease: the denial of one factor or the opposite of the coincidental oppositorum. This is why Dualism remains a valid philosophy. The maximum types of dualism try to unite the opposites in a kind of discern-ground dating. Each outcome is the opposite for every has the negative shape of the alternative. We cannot deny that the sector affects the mind, for sensory entry from the sector makes up most of the contents of the thoughts. We additionally can't deny that the mind outcomes the sector, for it animates a frame whose arms are adept at manipulating bodily truth.

But should we no longer just say that the body exits the arena immediately, without speaking approximately the hidden thoughts that govern it? Can we no longer say that a pc computes its input without having to define a ghostly laptop thought that reviews the qualia of its computational manner from within? It might be smooth to accomplish that if we had been no longer ourselves subjective beings, whose immediate experience of Being turned into no longer vital for the concept of Mind in the first place. Quantum Physics also casts doubt on the staunch materialist role by way of demonstrating the Observer Effect, whereby the mere presence of a watching mind changes the very material of ways light behaves. But this is no grounds for denying the frame. If our frame gets broken, we revel in pain, and that is sufficient evidence for me that the frame is actual, or ought to as a minimum be dealt with 'as if it was actual.

So what is the solution to this unsolvable dilemma? Like all dilemmas, we have to keep in mind that the fallacy arises from an oversimplification of a grand system, the maximum of which is past our capacity to realize. What originated first, the former and the latter. The solution of the route is neither. Chickens and eggs are both the same organism, and they passed off through a gradual process of evolution from which emerged all those characteristics that outline chickens, such as their oviparous nature. Even this answer is probably wrong as it accounts handiest for the knowable international, whereas the deep truths of the universe belong to the hidden world and are probably unknowable through the constrained processing power and lifespan of an organism residing inside that universe.

So with final reality perhaps all the time unknowable, we are left with pragmatism, which is the hallmark of Science. We roll with anything that works exceptionally to attain our ends, and for the method-whereby, we assume practical reality best inside the context of the application. To a neurosurgeon, the expertise of the mind in isolation is enough to get the process performed. A psychiatrist may additionally disregard the physical mind altogether and look alternatively at certain elements of body chemistry. To a standard health practitioner, all the organ systems have to be taken into consideration. To a holistic healer, all components of the individual from the physical through the emotional and ethical interplay with one another. To a medical psychologist, temper and behavior are both legitimate contexts in which to version someone. A motivational speaker tries to cope with people as intellectual centers of inertia. The point is that closing reality isn't knowable to us, and so our questions run away from us down paths described with the aid of epistemological fallacy. In truth, for you, truth is whatever you want it to be to get the job completed well. As for fact in itself, we can expect it exists due to the fact something must be casting those shadows at the cave wall. Study the shadows in some way you want to version them with the purpose to produce an era. Whether you need to version the arena as a singularity, a duality, or a more multiplicity, in terms of the product, the reality is the one that is 'accurate enough. The categories of concept with which we procedure data belong to us, to humanity, and though we're a part of the world, we aren't the sector itself. We should no longer be so foolish as to look for the Absolute using light human reason. To a certain point, it is unverifiable.

Chapter two

Your brain whilst you revel in trauma.

Trauma can have lots of outcomes in the mind. I've examined how it adjusts the development and structure of the mind, but I don't consider something particular about brain morphology. It also triggers a spread of coping mechanisms that the psychiatric profession calls "issues" but I think that's a huge misunderstanding. Trauma can motivate severe disorders, so to call coping mechanisms that assist you in function and continue to exist "issues" looks as if a huge mistake, to me in my opinion, trauma-induced me to dissociate. Additionally, it appears to have precipitated me to break up into some personalities, every of which protects all the different personalities in a few ways. I have separate components that do the following jobs independently and (until currently) without the understanding of every other part:

Take punishment, each physical and verbal. So, as an instance, when a person is indignant with me, this element comes to the front to take the punishment, and the relaxation of us don't have a good deal of reminiscence of the punishment. This has the benefit of saving us pain (even though the element has the unenviable job of storing the reminiscence of the pain), however, the disadvantage is that the rest of us can't learn from the enjoyment because we don't forget it. This is why we assume that punishment is a simply ineffective manner of modifying different human beings' behavior.

Analyze things severely. This element keeps watch over the entirety I/we do, and it looks for each form of failure that it could discover. This has the benefit of preparing us to fulfill the criticisms of other human beings, but the downside is that we never sense excellence about ourselves, or worthy of affection or attention. In addition, we don't ever experience as we matter. People often interpret that as low self-esteem and annoyingly try and urge us to sense better, unknowingly confirming that something is desperately wrong with us.

Analyze matters from a distance. This component has a unique attitude. It attempts to see things as objectively as feasible as if it can see matters from a godlike angle. It separates itself from our private hobbies and attempts to see matters from everyone's attitude. This is useful for empathy and verbal exchange and the matters this part says now and then strike others as "smart." However, this part has difficulty being sympathetic to ourselves or taking a subjective point of view, and it frequently makes it difficult for us to advise ourselves, leaving us quite at risk of being taken advantage of by manipulative human beings, especially those who aren't consciously manipulative.

Be innovative. There are numerous dissociated innovative elements. The major one is musical, however, there may be the person who makes use of physical intimacy to trigger resourceful visions of other worlds or ability realities, as properly. These components are capable of having a lot of amusing and being absolutely within the waft of what's happening, and we feel best whilst this sort of component is leading. Unfortunately, whilst that is not the case, we experience bereft and indignant loss. Also, these elements require the cooperation of other human beings to be innovative (bandmates or sexual companions or pals) and for the reason, that connection they require is as an alternative deeper than the general public is comfortable with, these elements require a splendid deal of protection and safety earlier than they're inclined to come to the front and do their aspect. This protection level is hard to offer for them, for the reason that trauma makes it extremely not likely we will believe anyone, and so we are constantly lonely and depressed and frequently come to suppose lifestyles are simply too difficult while those elements fall into despair approximately ever locating human beings they could thoroughly play with. People constantly are available and out of our lives, and these parts develop attached speedy (possibly too quickly) and despair fast whilst matters move wrong (again, possibly too speedy), and this conduct is what we've given us a bipolar analysis (which we think is best the smallest a part of the behavioral demanding situations we face.

Feel feelings. One element turned into created to experience matters, in particular sadness. He took all of the sadness, leaving us unwilling or not able to cry or experience a great deal of the feelings he took. He had to do this to go away from us capable of the feature. Emotions are very debilitating for us. We can not make selections or take motion if we feel emotions. But then, when we don't experience emotions, our moves and choices are made without information about our feelings, and that's also a hassle. We are true at pretending to be a socially perfect individual whilst this part hides our feelings from us, however, we're not able to make emotional connections because different people sense we aren't sincerely present.

Store the memory of the trauma. Until very currently, one part had the only activity of remembering what came about and keeping it a secret from the relaxation folks. One person was by chance visiting the "basement" (of our psyche) and noticed this component lurking in a dark nook, and we foolishly requested the element what it was doing. Firstly, we weren't even certain if it was among us. It could have been from somewhere else. But we requested what it turned into. It asked us (smiling a malicious smile) if we have been positive we desired to recognize. We foolishly said sure, and for the reason that then, the reminiscence of the trauma has been slowly discovered in a sequence of flashbacks. We don't like naming the trauma, except when we're irritated, and by some means, being requested approximately trauma makes us angry, so we can say it turned into a rape. We have been raped. I turned into raped. I became an "I" at the time. The rape caused a few large dissociations and the splitting off of numerous elements. However, the ability to break up this manner was installed region years earlier through some other activities, including unintentional occasions and deliberate events introduced on through the parenting theories of our parents. The part with the memory is now allowing us to get admission to the reminiscence, and the relaxation folks don't accept as true when it came about. We believe the part while we feel the flashback, however afterward, we really can't apprehend how that part ought to have kept that a secret these kinds of years. Everything that comes about in our lives makes a lot of sense in light of the trauma, however, we certainly can not keep in mind it happening personally, and so we all doubt that it certainly happened.

These are the diverse kinds of dissociation that our mind uses to help the character (or humans) on this body live on. Without the dissociation, we would have been hugely dysfunctional, and possibly would have died, both by accident or on motive, or, at a minimum, have been institutionalized and drugged right into a stupor, and by no means controlled to do whatever in existence.

We can see, functionally, what the dissociation did in phrases of conduct, the splitting into elements that assumed different roles, and the lack of know-how of the alternative parts and their roles. As an effect, we frequently discovered ourselves to have executed things we didn't consider doing and couldn't recognize what had stimulated us to do the one's matters. We agree that we're liable for the entirety our frame did, even supposing we weren't aware of choosing the one's actions at the time we performed them.

We also agree that there had been bodily changes to our mind shape and features that came about because of the trauma to facilitate dissociative coping strategies. We do not suppose this stuff is an issue or ailment. We assume they are hit adaptations to trauma.

These adaptations in reality have plus facets and poor facets. We aim to decrease the poor, at this point in existence. We don't understand how capable we're of doing that, but we feel that stepped-forward communication among the elements is vital to enhance consequences. We aren't in any respect certain we can be able to get what we want in lifestyles if we're sincere about ourselves. We don't assume all people will believe us sufficiently to be intimate with us. We don't suppose we can agree with anybody sufficient to, well, permit us to rely upon them. We're screwed, we assume, and so melancholy is a steady associate.

How does the brain address trauma?

It does what it could to live to tell the tale.

The Ego works to undergo defense mechanisms. The wholesome Ego can in reality be hurt, so move easily on humans. All people.

But deeper hurts can trace the development of the brain. The mind is likewise regarded to be elements and portions or zones, every with features, and as they overlap, damage or any form of birth illness could make the man or woman at risk of change. Neuroplasticity is a kind of defense mechanism of variation for survival. However, the mind has its primitive parts and can make mistakes and overdo them.

Shock or contamination in cardiovascular fall apart is a physiologic analog to this, while it, too, overdoes it to make amends for damage along with bacterial contamination (sepsis). It is going a long way and the patient can die from a cascading collection of primitive reactions or too many reactions completely.

When it comes to emotional trauma, one desires to recognize that it's far a conflict for survival through a person's resilience and the depth of the emotional trauma. One character's problem tolerating insults is every other character's life-changing harm. Battling those - either with trouble or ease are capabilities one acquires and will become greater resilient without being a hard-ass. Bruce Lee stated, "Do not pray for an easy life - pray alternatively for the energy to undergo a tough one."

In a way, you could pass back, or heal, in present-day theories that have recuperation powers and equipment for the and should IMO. By going back, I mean reconciling with dad and mom if it's far possible if this is where the resentment came about. The key isn't to address modern realities and to delete the beyond a few human beings who try to the abandonment of their own families as though to assist. Does it? I note that an evaluation of the past for a deeper understanding of what in reality occurred rather than 'handling' what one felt passed off allows the man or woman to participate greater in their care. I don't agree with that abandoning dad and mom because they deserve it or that the reality is that they'll never care; I believe they do care and that the child does now not recognize that; they may hurt as a whole lot as the kid does; the character with BPD was wrong in taking flight or rejecting them, in large part because they misread dad and mom. Tons of youngsters try this; some kids cannot navigate it at all. I never thought that accepting the 'fact' that one is unwanted is a great fact remedy. It isn't. Too often in psychology, the affected person is downright mistaken, and the 'trade' that the affected person and therapist seek together might be inclined to just accept exchange? Is to correct the wrong experience, to restore capacity and autonomy in the man or woman, and to live in fact and solve real troubles instead of delusional ones and get nowhere rather than seeking to somehow be given the fallacious notions as unchangeable.

Does trauma rewire the brain?

Great question. Normally human beings don't see that the changes suffered all through traumatization that gets bolstered after the event is gone using staying in a kingdom of panic, defeat, and hopelessness, and are certainly reprogramming the mind.

The rewiring that takes place because of traumatization has to do with preserving the brain working in 'survival mode' the use of emergency mechanisms that regulate the manner our mind and frame have to be regularly running.

All circuits become automated while they're repeated and used constantly due to the fact the brain assumes that the brand new circuit is going to be wanted, and therefore, it learns it. Every time the circuit is used, the more potent it becomes.

That's what trauma is: a new application, a mal-version. software that keeps the frame shooting stress hormones and looking forward to threats anywhere in a very subjective manner. A new application that 'learned' to be suspicious of everybody and the whole lot. A new 'addiction' that maintains disconnecting neurons to keep away from aches. A poor and ineffective manner to use the energy of the mind to avoid loss of life even if there is not even hazard.

Your brain completely changes with each life experience let alone trauma. Your neurons constantly adjust the synapses to house new data so that you can recognize that co-employee in your new task, keep in mind that paragraph in that aspect of the page of that book in the exam and plenty greater paraphernalia that you can list right now.

What is extra, although it sits encased within the thick protection of the skull, this three-pound jelly of flesh can undergo permanent alteration. This is pathological.

Chapter three

Trauma Symptoms

There are diverse methods trauma can affect an individual and this comes with special signs and symptoms relying on how your body translates the results.

What are the symptoms of trauma in Youth?

- They experience guilt for doing matters for their pleasure and happiness.
- They'd alternatively die than say 'no' to a person they don't need to lose.
- They sense as if they must make absolutely everyone around them happy.
- They're massive human beings pleasers.
- They don't proportion their issues due to the fact they don't want to be a burden on anybody else.
- They're too precise at faking happiness.
- They get induced effortlessly, however, are mannered to compress the ones that caused feelings.
- They tend to run far away from individuals who show comparable trends as their abuser did.
- They get plenty of pretty naturalistic nightmares and take days to forget about the info.
- They experience like they're faking it and there's been no trauma by any means.

- They get annoying effortlessly.
- They continue to be in poisonous situations trying their best to show a circle into a rectangle.
- They punish themselves when things go wrong.
- Not relying on what they gain, they nearly usually experience worthlessness and a burden to the arena.
- They can demise of pain however they receive shed a tear until they're positive no one's looking.
- They look 'ordinary' and 'wholesome'.

Note- All these symptoms aren't for everybody, all of us undergo matters in a different way.

Other Symptoms of Trauma Include:

- Persistent avoidance such as emotions, thoughts, and conditions
- Re-experiencing the trauma which might also contain flashbacks, nightmares, and distress while reminded of the event
- Negative changes in temper and thinking – that may purpose emotions of

numbness, blaming others or oneself, less interest in activities, or feeling detached from truth

- Changes in reactivity and arousal range include irritability, aggressiveness, sleep issues, problem concentrating, and reckless behavior.

In addition to drug addiction, alcoholism, and despair, the prognosis of PTSD regularly co-occurs with anxiety and consuming disorders.

What are Different Types of Trauma?
PTSD

PTSD, or Post-Traumatic Stress Disorder, happens when, many months after the worrying event, someone continues to be stuck in survival mode. They were not able to manage their recollections, and maintain to operate even though they are at risk. At this point, the neurological and hormonal adjustments aren't acute but continual. Physiological changes have occurred for the duration of the frame, affecting the functioning of all body structures.

When the anxiety and pressure from a stressful event will become continual and notably disrupts the manner someone lives, the man or woman can be recognized with PTSD. PTSD takes place while the frame's regular mental defenses in opposition to pressure become overwhelming. There is a substantial disorder with the normal defense structures after the trauma, which causes sure symptoms. This is why the regular recommendation for combating insomnia, anger/mood management, anxiety reduction, and so on., do no longer paint a person with PTSD. By the time someone qualifies for a prognosis of PTSD, the symptoms are not mental. They are physiological and systemic. At that factor, pointers which are based on changing one's attitudes or behavior are useless.

One of the primary motives a person can also expand PTSD in preference to being able to method their trauma is due to the fact they don't have their love and belonging wishes met. An individual can also enjoy trauma and then pass back to an empty house night after night, with nobody to share their studies with. They may fit lower back to a family who doesn't know the trauma took place, does not even accept it as true when it passed off, or would not accept the individual that experienced the trauma and the way it modified them.

Others won't have any stability or protection at home, may be out of labor or not able to preserve a process, and be missing their fundamental safety wishes. They might not have their bodily and health needs met. The paintings of processing trauma can not be effortlessly completed, and someone who is nevertheless simply seeking to survive can not do much to move out of survival mode related to the beyond.

Acute Stress Disorder

Acute Stress Disorder shares many similarities with PTSD. However, it's far from identified when symptoms were given between three and thirty days. Symptoms of acute pressure disease include stressful recollections, feeling indifferent, issues with concentration, avoidance, and a bad temper. People with acute pressure ailment can also experience a lot of guilt about not preventing the trauma or for no longer being able to circulate from it quickly.

Developmental Trauma

Developmental trauma describes a wide variety of destructive events that take place throughout early life, inclusive of abuse (sexual, bodily, or emotional), rejection, betrayal, being deserted, or witnessing demise or violence. Individuals who revel in developmental trauma have an improved chance of growing intellectual health situations which include PTSD.

Complex PTSD

Complex PTSD is a term that often describes the results of numerous reviews of developmental trauma. Survivors of those studies may also have deeply rooted poor beliefs approximately themselves or even the arena. They are used to being in a method of survival. They regularly fluctuate between feeling numb and excessive emotional states and are overwhelmed using their feelings. It is likewise commonplace for people with Complex PTSD to consider that no person is aware of them.

How To Know If a Person Develops Trauma?

Even though the signs and reasons for trauma vary, there are some common signs of trauma that others can appear. People who've experienced annoying occasions commonly seem disoriented and shaken. They may also have a hard time responding to communication as they could typically and regularly seem withdrawn or distant, even if they may be talking.

Another telling sign of a sufferer of trauma is anxiety. Anxiety because of trauma can motivate issues along with irritability, edginess, temper swings, bad awareness, and night terrors. Even though these signs and symptoms are pretty commonplace, they're not all-inclusive. People reply to trauma in various ways.

Sometimes even friends and family contributors cannot tell that a loved one is stricken by trauma. That is why it is critical to speak to someone following a disturbing event, even supposing they no longer display any signs of disturbance. In truth, it may take days, months, or even years for trauma to manifest following the real occasion.

If someone has PTSD from an early life trauma and is traumatized again later in life, do they go through the identical signs and symptoms as the first time or can their symptoms emerge as worse?

They tend to link and synergize. They develop and pick up different insecurities. That's why getting them healed quicker in place of later is counseled. The entanglements of the jungle worsen. Many of the demanding activities I've needed to deal with from military to vehicle wrecks have returned to some feeling of helplessness, hopelessness, and depression at some time once they had been an infant. That's why sometimes the latest occasion is not that bad and they are aware of it but it nevertheless has spun them off into melancholy, tension, or each other. So sure, they do connect and make things worse.

To heal those, therapists have devised specific fashions or techniques. They all work however I have located a few work way better than others and a few have precipitated extra trauma in the try to make it higher.

There is the don't forget each detailed institution that assumes you have to keep in mind each shred of worrying memory.
There are the repeat groups who make you relive it time and again until you do not care any greater.
There is the suck it up and be thankful for your alive institution.
They distract you with exhilaration.
There is the share with others who have long passed via its group.

There is the use of alcohol or capsules.

There is an organization that believes slicing or self-harm helps.

There is the use remedy from the prescription group.

There is the flip it over to God and don't worry about it.

There are the simply forget it organization (that is the maximum popular).

There is the guided imagery institution who has you create a special outcome.

There is the reverse timeline organization that sucks the power out of it.

There is the organization that creates a secure region to in the end speak approximately as soon as the individual can then permit it to pass and circulate on.

Each of these has benefits, but helpers tend to use the only they discovered worked for something hard of their existence so task the remedy at the soul. Sometimes it works, a whole lot of instances do not. The wrong style for the specific affected person.

Since our thoughts work by using associations, especially unconsciously, it can get quite debilitating over the years. Some ways have positioned the demons to relax permanently but some complex factors allow for that. It is important to recognize that it's far feasible but many already wounded humans find it too annoying to type out an excellent therapist when they are stuck within the grip of put-up demanding flashbacks.

But the most essential thing to remember is that there are folks who are very skilled at helping others through the types of matters lurking deep in your vault. They can assist shine a few compassionate lights down there and change that darkness into mild. Just don't give up. There is hope to be had.

Emotional Trauma Symptoms

Trauma normally manifests through emotion, together with emotional symptoms like anger, denial, emotional outbursts, and unhappiness. Trauma sufferers may redirect their overwhelming feelings toward pals, their family participants, and other assets.

Physical Trauma Symptoms

A bodily manifestation of trauma is also not unusual. Common bodily signs and symptoms of trauma may include fatigue, lethargy, paleness, terrible attention, and a multiplied heartbeat. The victim may additionally experience panic assaults or tension. They can also have a tough time coping with certain conditions. The bodily signs and symptoms of trauma can be as real as signs of an infection or physical damage.

Generally speaking, physical trauma is greater than mental trauma.

Physical trauma is extreme harm to the frame. It is something you can see.

Blunt force trauma. When an object or force strikes the frame, frequently causes concussions, deep cuts, or broken bones.

Penetrating trauma. Whilst an object pierces the pores and skin or frame, commonly growing an open wound.

Psychological trauma is harmful to the thoughts that happen due to a distressing occasion. Trauma is regularly the result of an awesome amount of strain that exceeds one's potential to manage or integrate the emotions worried with that enjoyment.

Because we can not see psychological trauma it frequently gets taken much less critically than it should which could make the damage and struggling reasons worse.

Chapter four

Trauma Therapy Techniques.

The traumatic mind calls for trauma therapy
There isn't any single shape of trauma remedy that works for everybody, but it's far possible to find the proper method or mixture of techniques for each man or woman. Even though there are many one-of-a-kind techniques used at a trauma

treatment center, they all have the commonplace intention of integrating the traumatic occasion into the individual's life, instead of subtracting it.

Therapy assists you to integrate annoying event(s) and understand them which allows you to begin the restoration technique. Your reminiscences of the trauma will stay, however, they'll start to have much less energy over you and your emotions.

"Therapy is useful in regulating a person's feedback to the trauma they are feeling. It can offer them new talents to control their emotions and responses at the same time as also presenting a context and schooling around the event itself."

The following strategies are a number of the maximum common and powerful types of remedies that might be used at a residential trauma remedy center.

Trauma-Focused Cognitive Behavioural Therapy (TF-CBT)

Trauma-Focused Cognitive Behavioural Therapy (TF-CBT) is an evidence-based total treatment program that facilitates individuals to deal with the aftermath of a disturbing revelation. While CBT gives powerful methods for selling restoration and treating trauma-associated problems, TF-CBT makes use of a trauma-touchy technique and elevated strategies. The TF-CBT approach encourages customers to talk about their feelings and pursuits to assist humans who have experienced trauma discover ways to control hard or painful feelings more healthily.

Trauma-targeted CBT (TF-CBT) therapy is likewise a cognitive behavioral remedy in particular used for youngsters and young adults with trauma.

TF-CBT's purpose is to assist children to recognize false beliefs (which include who to blame for abuse), accurate unhealthy behavior patterns, and expanding new ways to cope, along with self-soothing and expressing their feelings. Parents or caregivers also are concerned with this approach.

A 2014 review trusted Source concluded that TF-CBT could effectively lessen symptoms of PTSD in a few kids, and the APA strongly recommends styles of CBT for treating PTSD.

Eye Movement Desensitisation and Reprocessing (EMDR)

Eye Movement Desensitization and Reprocessing (EMDR) is a trauma therapy developed by psychologist Dr. Francine Shapiro in 1987. The remedy is unusual in that it doesn't involve tons of speaking, it has ambitions to help your technique and launch disturbing reminiscences thru eye moves.

In an EMDR session, your therapist will ask you to preserve a selected thing of a disturbing occasion in mind while you recognize their hand shifting from side to side (or, on occasion, rhythmic tapping).

The intention is to help your brain "reprocess" the memory which wasn't fully processed at the time due to overwhelming stress by way of engaging each facet of your brain (called bilateral stimulation).

This reprocessing targets to release the reminiscences, in the long run relieving nightmares, flashbacks, and triggers.

For a few humans, EMDR might also yield effects faster than different types of therapy, which includes talk remedy.

A 2014 look by Shapiro discovered that 80% to 90% of humans saw effects in the first 3 sessions, while a 2017 evaluation determined it to be just as powerful as a cognitive behavioral remedy (CBT).

Note that EMDR seems to work first-class for unmarried-occasion trauma, and it can now not be as effective for complicated trauma or complicated PTSD.

According to the APA, EMDR therapy is a conditionally encouraged treatment for PTSD.

EMDR classes observe a preset sequence of eight levels or steps. Treatment requires the person in trauma remedy or inpatient trauma treatment to mentally consciousness of the demanding enjoyment or negative idea at the same time as tracking the therapist's shifting finger or a transferring light with their eyes. In a few instances, auditory tones also are used. It allows humans to heal from symptoms related to demanding memories and improves misery by assisting them to view the occasion in a much less worrying manner. By comprising bi-lateral eye movements, the method enables the circulation of painful recollections from the forefront of the mind into the lengthy-time period of reminiscence.

Other beneficial trauma remedy strategies which might be frequently utilized in a residential trauma treatment center consist of:

Trauma Resiliency Model (TRM) Skills Building

TRM is a somatic, or frame-based, remedy that resets the disturbed nervous system of people laid low with trauma. Clients discover ways to watch and sing their frightened machine responses once they sense depression, harassment, or demands so that they may be able to stabilize themselves when those responses arise.

Mindfulness-Based Cognitive Therapy (MBCT)

MBCT helps humans mindfully recognize and end up in song with their terrible feelings, thoughts, and physical sensations.

Trauma Releasing Exercises (TRE) Yoga

TRE yoga helps launch stress or tension that is associated with trauma via physical games that launch 'brought about' muscle tissues because of a tight or flight reaction. In reality, these muscle masses often remain shrunk till the preliminary trauma has been resolved.

Group Therapy

There are many exceptional groups of human beings coping with trauma. Both therapists and peers can lead group sessions. Some awareness of giving help at the same time as others serve an educational purpose. Group therapy is most effective when it's used in combination with a man or woman remedy.

Prolonged publicity therapy

Prolonged exposure (PE) is a behavioral remedy for PTSD that, as the name suggests, entails confronting the source of your fear to reduce anxiety around it.

Avoidance is an outstanding symptom of publish-disturbing pressure. PE remedy objectives to help you triumph over avoidance that evolved after your trauma.

During remedy, you'll learn how to manipulate your breathing, talk about your trauma, and gently confront your worry in the real world. For instance, a person who lived thru sexual assault would possibly go back to the region in which it passed off to assist them to recognise that the trauma is no longer going on and that they're now secure.

"The higher we despise the emotions, mind, sensations, reminder, and pictures that are connected to our trauma, the worse the signs of trauma end up," explains Avigail Lev, PsyD, an authorized medical behavioral therapist, writer, and director of the Bay Area CBT Center in California.

"So the most analytical way of nursing trauma is revealing people to the emotions, mind, sensations, reminiscences, locations, and pic related to their trauma because this aids in the technique of desensitization."

Somatic remedies

Traumatic reminiscences are held within the frame in addition to the thoughts. Somatic remedy specializes in how your feelings can physically impact the frame. These feelings can resurface all of a sudden if you stumble upon a trigger or something that reminds you of a trauma.

Somatic therapy ambitions to "launch" pent-up trauma to alleviate mental fitness symptoms and continual ache, the usage of methods which include developing frame attention and grounding to your frame.

A 2017 study by Trusted Source discovered that somatic experiences speak beyond traumas while exploring the frame's physical responses and sensations turned into a powerful treatment for PTSD.

Psychodynamic remedy

In psychodynamic remedy, your therapist will help you apprehend how your beyond has affected your present-day emotions, behaviors, and courting patterns.

The intention is that it will help you understand the subconscious reasons that power your behavior.

Your therapist may additionally help you apprehend how early adolescence studies, circle of relatives dynamics, and cutting-edge relationships which can be formed by using trauma affect your modern coping techniques and ideals about the arena.

According to a 2008 review, psychodynamic tactics in trauma therapy can lead to:

improved self-esteem

the usage of extra beneficial coping techniques, and less unhelpful coping strategies

advanced relationships

higher social functioning

The author says that psychodynamic methods may be particularly beneficial in treating complicated PTSD.

Additional treatments and techniques that let you heal from trauma include:

Accelerated resolution therapy

The Substance Abuse and Mental Health Services Administration (SAMHSA) recognized increased decision therapy (ART) as an evidence-based treatment for trauma-associated disorders in 2015 Trusted Source.

The method aims to help you find remedies from trauma quicker than different remedies for PTSD by supporting you "reprogram" how your mind stores your traumatic recollections in a single to a few classes. ART builds on other strategies, which include EMDR.

Hypnotherapy

Hypnotherapy is a famous alternative for human beings who have struggled with other remedy sorts, like EMDR or CPT.

In hypnotherapy, the therapist places you into a trance-like stance, where you're wide awake and aware, however comfortable and able to shut out distractions. Then, they work to lessen the emotion attached to the occasion.

"It can help free the emotional restraint of trauma because it brings the subconscious fears, mind, and reviews to a conscious level," explains Maria Micha, psychotherapist, and scientific intellectual health counselor.

"People can't get the right to channel their subconscious mind and alter the fear that is identified on that stage. Techniques which include hypnotherapy can help launch and replace the worrying revel in with practical questioning and mental patterns," she provides.

Narrative therapy

The narrative remedy is a more recent remedy approach in which your therapist will help you "re-creator" your tale to give your stories meaning and form how you see yourself and the arena you live in.

This method may want to help with various mental health problems. It permits you to task beliefs you maintain approximately yourself following trauma, which includes feeling "damaged" or powerless to exchange your instances.

Internal circle of relatives systems (IFS) is

a form of speech therapy evolved by using therapist and educator Richard Schwartz, Ph.D.

The idea holds that your persona incorporates special "elements," each with its traits. All elements are held using the "Self," or your center focus. So, like your own family has distinct participants, your persona has one-of-a-kind components, too, and all of them want what's high-quality for themselves.

Your therapist will help you get to understand your distinctive elements throughout classes. Some elements may be more stricken by trauma than others. The goal is to understand why some components are hurting and learn how to help them with compassion as opposed to forgetting about or exiling them.

Art and song remedy

Art therapy can assist improve intellectual fitness and guide recuperation from trauma. It can take many forms, inclusive of dance, drama, music, writing, and innovative art.

"I find artwork remedy very helpful in trauma therapy as the unconscious thoughts will regularly reveal the effects of the apprehensive pattern," explains Micha. "Clients are often surprised with the drawings they produce, as the art will screen suppressed subconscious feelings and fears. Music therapy, in the meantime, can recognize supporting human beings to ground themselves by way of writing songs or compositions to create affirmations and modify their thoughts or feelings. Musical spontaneity can help customers nonverbally survey unpleasant stories as the speech center of the brain can shut down at some stage in a demanding flashback," explains Kyle Fleming, a board-certified track therapist and founding father of a mental health exercise in Illinois dedicated to this kind of remedy.

Inner child work

Also called inner baby recuperation, inner baby paintings are a therapy that could help you heal from youth trauma. For example, Micha generally uses it towards the end of trauma therapy with a customer.

It involves "going in touch" together with your internal child's trusted Source to sense the way you felt at diverse ages and running to heal your inner child's wounds by creating the safe, comfortable inner and outer environments you needed as an infant.

"It can help human beings triumph over any emotions of guilt or disgrace they'll be protecting from youth," explains Jessica Pedersen, a licensed and certified clinical hypnotherapist.

Trauma systems therapy

Like trauma-targeted CBT, trauma systems therapy (TST)Trusted Source is designed for youngsters, teenagers, and young adults.

This remedy emphasizes the individual's emotions and actions. It additionally considers the position that threatening social surroundings or systems of care can play in preserving a younger man or woman in a dysregulated country.

Chapter 5

Healing from Trauma

If strain, tension, and other issues following a demanding event are affecting your lifestyle, it's important to look for an intellectual health professional or health practitioner as soon as feasible. The following movements also are useful as acquire remedies for trauma:

Learn approximately Trauma and PTSD:

Knowing greater approximately your circumstance facilitates you to recognize why you're feeling the way you're in addition to creating powerful coping strategies.

Do no longer Self-medicate

Using pills or alcohol to numb what you're feeling is far from healthful, even though it can appear tempting. Additionally, it can intervene with treatments you're receiving from a trauma remedy center and get in the way of actual healing.

Spend Time with Others

Spending time with those who care about and assist you helps you heal, even if you do not speak about what took place. Simply sharing time with those who love you gives incredible comfort.

Find a Support Group

Ask a therapist or intellectual fitness professional to help you discover a support institution or seek an online one at your place.

Seek Help at a Trauma Treatment Centre

Even though you might not feel the advantages of therapy properly, a remedy at a residential trauma treatment center can be effective. Remember that many people make a successful recuperation and that these items take time. Follow your trauma treatment plan and brazenly communicate along with your therapists or mental fitness experts.

If you or someone you care about is experiencing trauma or PTSD, then touch The Dawn today to get hold of a no-responsibility evaluation and analyze extra approximately how we allow you to. You can also call us on one of our toll-unfastened numbers.

Learning to inhabit your body

How do I connect with my body

Hatha yoga is good for making you reflect on consideration and higher admiration, the exceptional elements of your bodily shape. Modern managed gymnasium exercising can do the identical thing. Running instantaneous will make you an awful lot extra privy to your heart, lungs, and legs.

Listen to it. Trust that your thoughts approximately align along with your frame. **Meditate.** Close your eyes and feel your frame with every breath you're taking.

Meditate, because you're still and quiet and your mind can music to what your body desires and stay a healthy lifestyle and drink masses of water and get lots of sleep and don't do pills

Picture your frame. Picture your frame precisely how it feels internal. Listen to what your body tells you that you need after which you do it.

One most important way we will connect to the frame is through breath. By sitting, connecting with breath, counting in-breath and out-breath, noticing where its actions, in which it remains caught, how long it lasts, how you feel … this is the easiest way I recognize to connect to the frame.

And when you begin and continue working towards that space, there are numerous other approaches to deepen the relationship. But regrettably, breath is constantly first and last.

Letting move beyond may be tough. Events that people find difficult could have a significant effect on their lifestyles, from their ideals to the selections they make.

Some examples of past activities that can be hard to allow go of encompassing:

intimate relationships

perceived successes or screw ups

errors or regrets

occasions that had been frightening or demanding

However, there are ways to cope with the lingering effects of past stories. This may also involve training self-compassion, attempting mindfulness as a manner of specializing in the prevailing moment, or searching for a remedy to explore unresolved emotions.

Life stories affect people in a ramification of ways. Some human beings locate it easy to transport after a tough experience, whilst others discover that those reviews have an enduring impact on their intellectual health.

People who conflict to permit a cross of unique activities from the beyond may also have experienced trauma. Trauma is a form of the mental wound which can result from any distressing revel including loss, change, or deep embarrassment.

Often, humans accomplice trauma by being worried about a violent event, which includes conflict. However, it may affect all of us. The distress caused also can affect how humans think.

Some people experience rumination, or a tendency to assume excessively about the same matters. According to a piece of writing within the American Psychological Association's Monitor on Psychology, people who ruminate frequently have a history of trauma and believe that ruminating helps them gain insight.

However, rumination may additionally virtually make it harder to clear up troubles, thereby stopping human beings from transferring forward. It is a commonplace characteristic of depression, obsessive-compulsive ailment, generalized anxiety disorder, and submit-traumatic strain ailment (PTSD).

People can also hold onto the beyond for other motives. For example, they may long for superb studies that are now over or live on beyond activities due to a subconscious desire to avoid being hurt in the future.

How to let go of the past

The following steps may additionally assist people to start to flow on from troubling recollections, consisting of beyond errors or regrets.

Make a dedication to allowing pass

The first step towards letting move is knowing that it's far necessary and feeling equipped to do so. This can happen in distinct instances for special humans, but once someone makes this selection, it may be empowering.

Feel the emotions

Memories of beyond events can deliver complicated or strong emotions. Allowing oneself to experience those emotions unconditionally, without seeking to combat or fix them, is a vital step towards processing what befell.

This can be tough, so it can assist to express these emotions in a safe vicinity, which includes in a journal, with a trusted pal, or with a therapist.

Take responsibility

If relevant, it can assist folks that sense guilt, embarrassment, or shame approximately the beyond to take obligation for or her function within the event. This does no longer imply blaming oneself, however really acknowledging what came about and taking ownership of past actions.

This can help humans experience less helplessness and feel that if they can take duty for the past, they can do the same for their destiny.

Practice mindfulness

Mindfulness is an ability that encourages human beings to the consciousness of what's taking place inside the present. This can assist those who warfare with rumination.

One 2016 paper suggests that folks that are extra aware revel in much less rumination and are much more likely to be compassionate and closer to themselves.

Some approaches to exercise mindfulness consist of:

noticing small joys, such as the flavor of a scrumptious meal or the warm temperature of the sun on the skin

spending time in nature, bringing interest lower back to the surroundings every time the thoughts wander

conducting mindful, creative pastimes, together with drawing or gambling musical gadgets

practicing mindfulness meditation

There are many approaches to meditation. Beginners trying mindfulness meditation can strive:

sitting someplace quiet, with no distractions

last the eyes and taking numerous deep breaths

that specializes in breathing in and exhaling whilst mind of the beyond arise, in reality allowing them for a second before returning the focal point to respiratory

This persistent process of returning to the existing is the basis of mindfulness. Some may additionally discover it beneficial to visualize their thoughts floating away, while others may favor repeating a phrase that reminds them of the prevailing.

Practice self-compassion

Self-compassion is when you take care of yourself with kindness, care, and overlook your shortcomings. People can exercise self-compassion with the aid of changing their self-communication. This involves noticing while their mind turns out to be vital and changing them with more forgiving options. Keeping a self-compassion journal may be a great way to exercise this talent.

How to let go of past relationships

It can be mainly tough to allow the passing of relationships, as human beings shape deep attachments with each other.

In addition to the above recommendations, humans can take extra steps to let go of dating, including:

briefly or completely limiting contact with ex-partners

lowering reminders of them, together with hiding them on social media

putting and respecting obstacles

spending time on self-care and personal increase that specializes in what is viable outdoor of the relationship

According to psychologist Dr. Gary W. Lewandowski, Jr., older research indicates that thinking about effective factors of a breakup might also assist limit emotions of loss. For example, after a court case ends, some human beings may be able to pursue new desires, such as visiting, getting a pet, or locating a new career.

People who have been in dangerous or abusive relationships may additionally require extra support with letting pass, as trauma bonding can arise. Trauma bonding refers to having a dangerous attachment to a person who has handled a person abusively.

How to let go of resentment

Feelings of unresolved anger, betrayal, and resentment are not unusual among those who struggle to permit go of a past occasion. Anger and resentment also can arise in the aftermath of trauma or as a related function of PTSD.

Some extra steps to take to manipulate this emotion include:

Expressing anger in a safe manner

Some human beings are hesitant about expressing anger. However, psychologist Dr. Howard Kassinove states that anger and aggression aren't equal. While anger is a sense and physiological kingdom, aggression includes taking motion on one's emotions frequently in a way that causes harm.

It is possible to express anger in a secure way. For instance, humans can try:

writing about their emotions on paper and then throwing it away

expressing their emotions via artwork, track, or different creative hobbies

engaging in workout or sports activities, along with walking conducting workout or sports, together with running

People with anger due to trauma or PTSD might also benefit from extra trauma treatments.

Being open to forgiveness

The subject matter of forgiveness is arguable among humans who have skilled wrongdoing, together with betrayal, injustice, or abuse.

However, the National Domestic Violence Hotline emphasizes that forgiveness does not imply condoning the harmful movements of others or accepting their apologies. Instead, forgiveness can imply accepting that someone's movements had been destructive while additionally letting move of anger with a view to advantage one's very own well-being.

It can take time to paint in the direction of forgiving others or forgiving oneself. It may involve processing emotional pain, information about what brought on it, and considering what it might take to forgive.

How to let go of control

Those who feel they want to control many elements of their lives might also do so due to the fact they want to trust themselves or others. They may additionally have had negative reviews that created a fear of uncertainty, inflicting them to feel that the only answer is to control occasions as much as possible.

Learning to let go of control can also contain:
Identifying why the need for control exists and exploring ideals surrounding what occurs if one "loses" manage

figuring out emotions or events that trigger the want to manipulate and taking into account ways to cope with them in a more healthy way practicing letting cross of manipulating in small, conceivable steps, which include means of delegating a project to somebody else

starting to make decisions primarily based on love, in preference to fear

Over time, this can help human beings show to themselves that they no longer want to control things so that they will be happy or resolve issues.

Tips to Help With Trauma Recovery

- Owing yourself
- Talk with others about the way you sense. Don't isolate yourself.
- Calm yourself. Try meditation or deep respiration physical games. Do physical activity, like taking walks or doing yoga.
- Take care of yourself. Get plenty of sleep. Eat a wholesome eating regimen. Drink sufficient water.
- Avoid the use of alcohol, capsules, and tobacco.

- Get back to your daily habit. Do the matters you would commonly do, even in case you don't sense adore it.
- Get concerned about your community. Volunteering is a great way to create a sense of which means.
- Get help if symptoms persist. Talk with a mental fitness professional.
- If you're looking to help a pal, concentrate and find out where they're inside the coping technique. Try to just accept their feelings and assist in any manner you could.